A Dermatologist's Case Book

by

Edward S. Peterka MD MS

authorHOUSE™

1663 LIBERTY DRIVE, SUITE 200
BLOOMINGTON, INDIANA 47403
(800) 839-8640
WWW.AUTHORHOUSE.COM

First published by AuthorHouse 07/20/05

ISBN: 1-4208-4321-4 (sc)
ISBN: 1-4208-4322-2 (dj)

Library of Congress Control Number: 2005905077

Printed in the United States of America
Bloomington, Indiana

This book is printed on acid-free paper.

FORWARD

One of the richest and most rewarding experiences you can have is to be allowed into the private office of a master clinician. This book gives you that entry into the office of a master dermatologist. It lets you look over his shoulder as he ponders the puzzling problems of itch, warts, and contact dermatitus.

Here you see a modern Sherlock Holmes at work, detecting unique causes which vary from cigarettes to beer, and from upholstery to fiberglass. Here you see patients who were cured only after close inspection of their clothing, their diet, their health, their environment, and their psyche.

Whether you be a first year medical student, an experienced physician, or an inquiring patient, you will enjoy and profit from this book of dermatologic sleuthing. It bubbles with humor, wisdom, and insight.

Looking over Dr. Peterka's shoulder will enhance your skill as a doctor. Looking over his shoulder, as a patient, makes you aware of the significance of every detail of your daily life, from your pet skunk to your favorite walk in the park. Finally, looking over his shoulder, as a gentle reader, brings you an awareness of what can happen to your skin and why.

We all thank Dr. Peterka for letting us into his office on a busy day. We've all seen and learned a lot about skin around us.

Walter B. Shelley, M.D., Ph.D., M.A.C.P.
Professor Emeritus of Dermatology
Medical College of Ohio
Toledo, Ohio

E. Dorinda Shelley, M.D.
Professor of Clinical Dermatology
Medical College of Ohio
Toledo, Ohio

CHAPTER I

Itch! Itch! Itch!

or

"How I Started My Practice from Scratch"

Whenever I walk into a room to see a new patient and after introducing myself, I always ask the questions: What sort of problem do you have? Why are you here?

Sometimes if it's a man and he has a sense of humor he'll say, "My wife brought me here because she's tired of my scratching, and so am I. I want to know why am I itching?"

As Sherlock Holmes would say, let the chase begin. Itching is not a simple problem to solve. I would say to you, "Play detective." Here then are some unusual stories from my casebook to answer that question, "Why am I itching?"

THE FIBERGLASS STORY: Many

years ago when I first began my practice in dermatology, I saw a lady who came in to see me with the chief complaint of itching.

I asked her, "How long have you been itching?"

"Oh, about two weeks," she replied.

"Do you itch all over or only in certain areas?" I asked.

"Well, mostly" she said, "my back and hips itch."

"Have you ever been free of itching since the itching began?" I inquired.

"No, not really," she replied.

"How bad is the itching?" I asked.

She said, "It's pretty bad. Sometimes I could just scratch and scratch, and then it gets even worse."

"Are you diabetic? Do you have a kidney problem? Do you have liver or gall bladder disease?" I asked. She answered, "No" to all the questions.

In the winter, in Illinois, many patients sometimes have what is termed the winter itch from dry skin. There is no winter itch in the summer in Illinois. The humidity is just too high.

"Do you have any animals? Are you taking any medication? Do you have any medical problems that you are aware of? Is anyone else in the family itching?" I asked. To all of the questions, she answered, "No."

When I examined her, she did not show any dermographism. This is an easy test to do. When the skin on a person's back is stroked, a red line like a wheal will show up. No dermographism was noted. Her skin reacted normally. Sometimes I check the underclothing for bleaches, detergents, or chlorinated odors that could cause irritation and itching. Her blouse felt prickly. Using a magnifying glass, I saw a sharp fiber. As a matter of fact, her blouse was full of glass fibers.

"Did you recently, within the past two to three weeks, launder your fiberglass curtains?" I asked.

A look of surprise came upon her face as she said, "Yes, I did." In the 1970's white fiberglass curtains were quite common.

"Well," I said, "you probably washed your blouse and underclothing along with your white fiberglass curtains

"Feel these fibers and look at them under the magnifying glass," I said.

"By gosh," she exclaimed, "that is fiberglass!"

"There is your answer," I said.

I told her to get rid of her entire clothing that she had put in the wash with the fiberglass curtains. She did and her problem was solved.

She went to the front desk to pay for the office visit, and I heard her complaining to the receptionist, "Three dollars!" A long time ago my office fees were very low.

I went to the front desk and said to her, "You know, you remind me of the farmer who went to an attorney to ask what constituted a legal barbwire fence. The attorney said that a legal barbwire fence was three feet high with three strands of wire and that would be three dollars please. If I got paid for what I did, sometimes I would never get paid at all. I get paid for what I know and not what I do." I gave her a sample lotion.

A wise dermatologist once told me, always give the patient something to take home, either a sample of a lotion, a cream, a prescription, or an instruction sheet so that the patient feels like they are getting something. I've never forgotten that lesson. Always give the patient something to take away.

A SECOND OPINION: A young Asian woman about thirty came to see me with the chief complaint of constant itching. Occasionally it was intense. At other times, the itching was mild, but some itching was always present. In taking her history, I asked the usual questions: Are you diabetic? Do you have a kidney or liver problem? Do you take any drugs? She answered "No" to all questions.

I asked about scabies, food allergies, about her general health, etc. and could find no clues. She was not losing weight. She seemed to be happily adjusted. Her itching did not appear to be psychological but it was driving her to distraction.

I was looking for a focus of infection such as a bacterial, a fungal, or a viral infection, such as: abscessed teeth, tonsils, sinuses, infected gall bladder, colon, or fungus infection of the feet or toenails. After doing all of the laboratory tests and the C-reactive protein test, there were no clues. There was no history of internal malignancy. The dermographism test was minimally positive. Treatment for scabies and taking oral antihistamines did not help.

Finally, I said to her, "Would you like to get a second opinion?"

I'll be the first to admit that I don't know everything and a new approach from another perspective might be helpful. One of my teachers in dermatology taught that if you came to a dead end and are still puzzled, start all over again. Act as though you are seeing the patient for the first time. I suggested that she get a second opinion, and we agreed to a referral at a major university. She was thoroughly re-examined and a suspicious node was discovered which on biopsy showed Hodgkin's Disease. Now Hodgkin's Disease is a lymphoma characterized by intractable itching. Subsequently she underwent surgery, x-ray therapy, and chemotherapy. After months of treatment, she was finally pronounced cured. Her itching had disappeared. She later became pregnant and had children.

Years later, I saw the patient's mother, and her mother told me, "You know, Dr. Peterka, I am eternally grateful to you for getting a second opinion. If you hadn't done that, my daughter would not be alive today, and I would not be a grandmother."

I replied that I really didn't do anything and that I felt I was a failure for not finding the cause myself.

"No matter," she said. "if it were not for your referral, she would not be here today."

Never hesitate to get a second opinion. The point of this story is seek and you shall find. If one never seeks, one shall never find.

THE BEER DRINKER'S LAMENT:

The next story is about an African American man who came in to see me because he was itching all over. He showed a red, blotchy macular rash that was very faint.

In taking his history and asking the usual questions for generalized itching, I asked him, "In your opinion, what do you think is causing your itching?"

"I think it is related to my drinking beer," he said. "When I don't drink beer, the rash disappears and I'm okay. But if I have a beer, it doesn't take very long before I start itching."

After advising him on the use of laundry detergents and inquiring about cold, heat, sweating, and other foods I told him to avoid drinking beer or alcoholic beverages for the next two weeks. In addition, he was to stay away from all foods containing yeast products. He was to watch his diet, especially his liquid diet, (i.e., beer and fermented liquor). Two weeks later, he came in completely clear. He told me that this was the longest time that he could ever remember that he was free of itching. He knew what his problem was and what was causing him to itch. He had solved the case for me.

In parting, he asked me, "Can I ever drink again?"

"I can't guarantee that you won't have a recurrence of the problem with certain foods, alcohol, or beer, but if you wish to use vodka, which is distilled and as close as you can get to pure grain alcohol, you could mix some vodka with orange juice, which is called a stinger. That may not sting you." I said.

In conclusion, these stories illustrate the fact that seeking the cause of a patient's itching is like playing detective (seek and ye shall find). Entire chapters of textbooks of dermatology are devoted to the causes of itching. Sometimes it is a real challenge.

An Asian woman came to see me and told me that she was itching "down below". What she really was saying is that she was having vaginal or rectal itching which can be very embarrassing. The itching may be the result of a variety of causes such as pin worms, parasites, a yeast infection, or unusual problems such as extramammary Paget's Disease and others. After asking the usual questions for causes of a yeast infection such as a history of recent oral antibiotics and diabetes and checking for symptoms of burning of the mouth and tongue or redness and itching in the inter-digital spaces, a physical examination showed a chronic vaginal yeast infection. A recent history of oral antibiotics supported the diagnosis.

The usual cause of a yeast infection is the organism Candida albicans. (Candida – Latin for small and albicans – Latin for white). The colonies on culture are small, round, and white

"What is the treatment?" she asked.

I replied, "A drug company recently came out with a new pill that is very effective. One pill will eliminate any vaginal yeast infection, but it is very expensive."

"Well, I can't afford a lot of expense," she grumbled.

"There are some less expensive drugs such as Mycostatin tablets or Mycostatin oral suspension," I replied.

She persisted, "I don't want to pay for anything that is expensive."

She was one of the most frugal patients that I had ever met

"You can go to the drug store and buy a vinegar douche that is already bottled," I replied.

She was like a dog after a bone and she persisted in asking, "Is there anything else that I can use?"

"Yes," I said, "you can take some water and put some vinegar in it. It doesn't matter if you use red, white, or apple vinegar, and you can make a douche. Furthermore, if you don't use it all up, you can add some oil to it and use it as a salad dressing. That way you won't be wasting anything." She took my advice, and made a homemade vinegar douche.

CHAPTER II

Location! Location! Location!

or

"How You Can Make the Diagnosis on the

Location of the Rash"

The location of the rash often leads to the diagnosis. Some diagnoses are quite simple to make, and one can make the diagnosis merely by observing where the rash is located. For example, a rash on the earlobes is most likely a contact dermatitis to earrings. However, a secondary infection may be present. There may be, in addition to an infection, a reaction to the topical that is used. If the rash is located at the lower back of the neck at the collar line of the clothing, the label may be the cause of the itching. Many labels contain India ink that cross-react to poison ivy. If the patient is allergic to poison ivy, he or she will react to the India ink in the label. If the rash is located on the top of the feet where the straps of a sandal rub, one should consider a contact dermatitis from the leather of the sandals or from the tongue of old tennis shoes. An old tennis shoe often completely wears out except for the tongue, which reminds me of some patients who are all worn out except for their tongue. At one

point in time, there was a rash (no pun intended) of

contact dermatitis from sandals made in India. In

many instances, the location of the rash will often

lead to the diagnosis. Books of dermatology have

been written on the distribution of skin rashes and

how to diagnose by location. These cases will

illustrate examples of diagnosis by location and the

pitfalls that occasionally may occur.

THE PET SKUNK: A number of years ago, a woman came to see me with a rash on the left side of her neck. The rash showed no distinguishing features. It was blotchy and faintly red. Complete skin examination from her scalp to her feet showed a rash only on the left side of her neck.

I wondered why the rash was present only on the left side of her neck so I asked her, "Is there something different that happens on the left side of your neck than anywhere else? Do you rub something on that area such as a cream or a perfume that you do not use on the right side of your neck? What do you do different on the left side of your neck?"

"Well, come to think of it" she said, "my pet skunk sits on my left shoulder."

"Is it descented?" I asked.

"Yes, he is," she replied, "but sometimes the fur of his underside is moist after he urinates."

"That is your answer." I said.

"What should I do?" she asked.

"Just keep the skunk off your shoulder and you'll be okay." I replied. The point of this story is to look for the unusual location of the rash.

THE ITCHY NIPPLES: In the early 1970's, jogging was the "in" thing to do especially with college students. Many of the coeds at the time went without a bra. Articles at the time cautioned about jogging without a bra as the friction from the tank top could cause an irritation of the nipples. Sometimes the detergents and bleaches in the tank tops could complicate the problem. A young Asian coed was seen in the office with an irritation quite evident on and around her nipples. I explained to her that she should start wearing a bra whenever she went jogging. I gave her a cream to help alleviate the reaction.

Several weeks later, she came in again and complained that the rash was still present, but not always. At times, it would clear up with the cream, and then later it would again recur. She insisted that she always wore her bra when she went jogging and throughout the day, so that it appeared that the contact dermatitis had been eliminated. Yet she still was having intermittent bouts of redness and itching involving her nipples. Without causing her embarrassment, I asked her, "Does your boyfriend suck on your nipples?"

"Yes, every so often." she replied.

"That is why you have the rash on your nipples." I said.

The yeast Candida albicans normally resides in the mouth and in the saliva, so that both contact irritant factors and a yeast infection caused her itchy nipples.

This same case study can be applied to those children or adults who lick their lips. This leads to chapping of the upper or lower lip which is characterized by dryness and peeling. This often is complicated by a yeast infection. There is a condition called perleche that occurs as an irritation at the angle of the mouth from the drooling of saliva at night when the patient is sleeping on that side. He or she will wake up with moisture in the angle of the mouth on one side or the other and occasionally on both. Another example of this same irritation can occur between the interdigital spaces or under a ring on the ring finger. This condition is given the exotic name of erosio interdigitalis blastomycetica. Nickel in earrings, necklaces, wristwatches, or rings may cause a contact dermatitis. Patients will say their jewelry is pure gold. There is no such thing as pure gold. Pure gold is too soft. Small amounts of nickel are added to harden it. Hypoallergenic earrings can now be bought that do not contain nickel. Stainless steel earrings worn in the ear lobes or stainless steel beads in the nose, tongue, and eyelids do not appear to cause a reaction. The steel is the type used in orthopedic surgery.

THE EYES HAVE IT: A problem seen in women often occurs on the eyelids or around the eyes. These women come in with various degrees of redness, dryness, flaking, and edema of the eyelids. Sometimes there is acute dermatitis and severe swelling and sometimes barely visible faint pink patches.

In taking the history, usually I ask, "Do you wear fingernail polish?" Nail polish is a common cause of this reaction.

I also ask, "Do you use eyebrow pencils, mascara, eyeliners, or eye shadow? Do you wear glasses? If so, how strong are they? Does your husband wear cologne or an after-shave lotion that might come in contact with the area around your eyes? I'm not saying that you should get rid of your husband, but be aware of the fact that something that he might be wearing may be causing you the allergic reaction.

In addition, a secondary yeast infection may also play a role in some cases. Airborne allergens such as pollens, molds, grasses, trees, chemicals, fertilizers, and dusts in the air may cause an allergic reaction. If the location of a rash is around the eyes, one should consider the more unusual causes such as dermatomyositis or photodermatitis. If a patient takes medication that causes photodermatitis and wears strong glasses, a rash may only occur around the eyes. An acne-type eruption around the mouth in a perioral distribution may appear as a reddish rash. In this instance, oily products and greasy moisturizers plug up the hair follicles causing a combination of acne-type lesions and dermatitis. The treatment is to avoid the heavy lubricants and to use a non-comedogenic moisturizing cream. A yeast infection may also enter into the mix as well as a bacterial infection. Pressure put on these areas from the palm of the hand or the knuckles is a contributing factor. Again, the location of the rash leads to the diagnosis. As in real estate and as in the diagnosis of a skin rash, location, location, location is one of the most important considerations.

CHAPTER III

Hives

or

"An Easy Diagnosis a Difficult Solution"

Most of the time the average layperson is able to make a diagnosis of hives. Hives are easily recognized, but the cause may not be so easily recognized. The sixty-four dollar question then becomes what is causing the hives? To answer the question what is causing the hives may not be easy.

Unless the cause is found, the hives will continue to

be a problem and will continue to plague the patient.

The solution is to find the cause of the hives, but the

solution may be difficult.

CASE OF THE MENTHOL CIGARETTES: Many persons smoke cigarettes.

Cigarette smoke contains carbon monoxide and smoking cigarettes is believed to be a cause of lung cancer. The smoke is offensive to many people, and in, general, cigarette butts are messy. A number of years ago, a woman with hives came to see me. In those days, a patient could be hospitalized and put in isolation. In this way, all of the possible causes of an allergic reaction from the environment such as perfumes, dusts, pollens, grasses, weeds, and other airborne allergens could be removed. The patient would be put into a room that was essentially bare of all furniture. Everything would be taken away except the hospital gown and a toothbrush. The diet was limited to cooked rice and bottled spring water. All visitors were prohibited. The nurses came in wearing a cap and gown as if the patient had some contagious disease and required isolation. The purpose of this isolation was to remove all outside allergens that could be causing the problem. If the patient continued to have hives, in spite of removing all of the outside environmental allergens, one could conclude that the cause of the hives was internal. If, after five days of isolation, the patient had no hives, then a search would be made for an internal cause of the hives. After five days of isolation, this patient had no hives. A battery of tests such as a complete blood count, urinalysis, C-reactive protein, blood chemistries, chest X-rays, ear, nose, and throat cultures were done. These were all negative. In the meantime, the patient was given some amenities such as smoking because most smokers begin having nicotine withdrawal after five days. After smoking a couple of mentholated cigarettes, the patient noticed an outbreak of hives. This was the first time that she had hives all the while she was in isolation. When she stopped smoking, she stopped having hives. It appeared then that she was allergic to smoking cigarettes. However, she discovered that she could smoke regular cigarettes without getting hives. One of the axioms in searching for the cause of hives is to look for two causes. Staying away from mentholated cigarettes and from smokers who smoked mentholated cigarettes solved her problem. The solution for her was to stick to regular cigarettes, and to this day she still smokes regular cigarettes. In her case, the problem was solved. It was the end of her hives.

THE DODGE COLT: This man presented

a puzzling case of hives. His hives were not present

on a daily basis. They were intermittent. Sometimes

he would get them at work but not always. There

was no particular pattern. He was hospitalized in

a similar manner and placed in isolation. He was

placed in isolation and isolated from all outside

allergens. He was given a thorough work-up and

no internal causes of his hives were found. While

he was in the hospital, he never had hives. The only

clue that appeared to be of significance was that his

hives always appeared at work. In questioning him

closely, he revealed that on some days after arriving

at work he had no problem. On other days, he had

severe hives shortly after he arrived at work. The question was what was causing the hives on that one day when he had them at work and not on the other work days when he had no hives. Finally, I asked him what was different about going to work when he got the hives after arriving at work and the days when he had no hives.

He thought a while and said, "Maybe it's the car I ride to work in. Some days I ride in a certain car, and I have hives shortly after I arrive at work. When I ride in another car, nothing happens."

"Well, which car do you ride in that seems to cause the hives?" I asked.

He said, "I think it's a Dodge Colt."

The Dodge Colt was a new car from Japan. It had a distinctive odor of new leather. I called the local Dodge dealer and asked him if he had a Dodge Colt on the showroom floor. Sure enough, he had one, and he was willing to do an experiment. He arrived at the hospital with a brand new Dodge Colt. The patient sat in the back seat. The salesman was the driver, and I sat next to him while we toured the countryside. The patient was quite happy because at least he was getting out of the hospital for a while and was enjoying the ride. We got back to the hospital and shortly thereafter he had hives. The next day we used a car other than a Dodge Colt. He had no hives after riding in that car. We concluded that the cause of his hives was the odor of the leather from riding in the Dodge Colt. If he did not ride in the Dodge Colt, he had no hives. When he found this out, he shot out of the hospital like a bullet from a Colt 45. He avoided a Dodge Colt after that and the problem of his hives was solved.

YOU CAN SWEAT OUT THE DIAGNOSIS: THE DRUM MAJOR STORY.

A number of years ago a drum major in a school band came in with a complaint of hives after marching in a parade. After listening to the description of his hives, it was clear that he had cholinergic urticaria. This type of urticaria can result from heat, cold, sweating, or a combination of heat and sweating. The test for cold urticaria is to put a square ice cube on the forearm, which then causes a square hive. This test is unique as one never sees a square hive in nature. The test for heat and sweating urticaria is to have the patient exercise. The heat, sweating, and the changes in temperature cause the reaction.

In this case, the young man was asked to walk up and down the stairwell of my six-story office building. After about the third trip up and down, he came back into the office with urticarial papules. This type of cholinergic urticaria is often difficult to treat. The patient is warned in the cases of cold urticaria to avoid cold drinks and jumping into cold water as this may trigger a histamine release and possible death. Since the papular urticaria happened only after he marched several hours at the head of the band, it was felt that oral medication such as cyproheptadine and hydroxyzine hydrochloride with an antihistamine could be taken before each parade. By the time he reached the end of the parade, he had enough of the medication in him to prevent

the allergic reaction from occurring. In this case,

the patient literally sweated out his hives which

was prevented by taking his medication before he

marched at the head of the parade.

CHAPTER IV

Warts! Warts! Warts!

or

"Warts Will Humble You"

Years ago when I first started teaching, I thought I would write a book on the treatment of warts. At the time, some 35 years ago, my secretary collected every known article on warts in the library that was published regarding the types of warts, their locations, their causes, and treatment.

Back then, I was able to find about 500 articles concerning warts. The conclusion of my research proved that there was no one treatment that would cure all warts. Some treatments worked for some patients, and other treatments worked for other patients. For the most part, however, most of the treatments did not work. This chapter will discuss some of the most interesting treatments that have been tried.

WARTS RESISTANT TO ALL

TREATMENT: Some warts are resistant to treatment no matter what you do. The most memorable case of this type of wart was a woman who developed warts on some of her toes. After all the treatments on her toes had failed, they were amputated. She then developed warts on the soles of her feet and stumps of her toes. Subsequently, she had an amputation at the ankle. The ankle stump developed warts so that it became extremely painful to walk with a prosthesis. Thinking that a below the knee amputation would remove the warts and allow for a solid prosthesis, such amputation was done. In spite of this radical treatment, she developed warts on the stump. She subsequently became so despondent that she committed suicide. In her case, the resistance of the warts to all types of therapy led to her despondency and her suicide. This was the worst case scenario that I had ever encountered.

Most warts will respond to some form of therapy, but not always. In the book <u>Tom Sawyer</u> the advice was given that if you want to cure warts, just soak them in skunk water from a hollow stump, and according to Huckleberry Finn, it worked every time. Some practitioners have tried to smother the warts by applying adhesive tape on a weekly basis. Using duct tape instead of adhesive tape recently revived this old form of treatment. In either case, the result is about the same. Some warts respond, and some do not. In a trial therapy of a 100 patients using adhesive tape, half of the patients were cured of their warts. What can be said of the adhesive or duct tape therapy is that it is economical, safe, and possibly effective. Certainly it is worth trying.

The treatment of warts using the psyche has been known for a long time. As to why this type of therapy works it is anybody's guess. Some researchers feel that the psyche has a direct effect on the vasculature of the wart. It is a well known fact that patients blush with embarrassment or turn white with fear. Those methods that appear to be successful may somehow affect the blood vessels

of the wart. The following are some examples of

the effect of the psychic on the warts.

SETTING THE WARTS ON FIRE:

This method seems to be most effective in younger children and definitely involves the psyche. The child is brought into a dark room. The warts are painted with fluorescein, and then a black light or Wood's light is used to fluoresce the warts. This causes them to glow bright red orange in color.

All the while the warts are being fluoresced, the practitioner intones in a deep low voice, "See, the warts are on fire. They are burning up."

As the young child's eyes grow large, the idea of the warts being burned up is suggested to the patient. After the treatment with the Wood's black light, the patient is told not to touch the warts. Two to three weeks later, the warts are gone. Hypnosis works in the same way. The therapist hypnotized the patient. In a post-hypnotic suggestion, the therapist tells the patient that every time he or she touches the wart they will feel an electric charge or current flow from their finger into the wart. The patient believes that this electrical current is slowly but surely destroying the wart. Warts have disappeared with post-hypnotic suggestion.

In some patients, I have treated the mother wart, which I define as the first wart that appears that is still present. This mother wart is treated, and often three weeks later, the other warts will have disappeared. In all of these cases, it appears that the power of suggestion somehow affects the vascular nature of these warts or the immunity of the patient. Those individuals who lack immunity, such as patients who have AIDS, have a sudden outbreak of numerous warts. One of the signs of AIDS in some individuals is the sudden appearance of warts. The immune system in many ways affects the health of the individual. Those with low immunity are subjected to a variety of diseases and infections. The role of immunity in warts is yet to be settled.

One of the treatments of warts is to cause a reaction in the wart itself. Applying a well-known sensitizer such as poison ivy to the wart can do this. However, using poison ivy could also lead to development of an allergy to poison ivy where otherwise it did not exist. Certain chemicals in nature that are never found can be used. These substances can be used to provoke an allergic reaction in the wart and therefore create immunity. The injection of Bleomycin, an anti-cancer drug, into the wart is an optional treatment. These drugs often result in some remarkable cures. In genital warts, podophyllin may be used to treat the warts.

After trying the numerous therapies such as electrodesiccation, cryosurgery, excisional surgery, fluorescent dyes, hypnosis, adhesive tape, duct tape, cantheridin, podophyllin, and the injection of

Bleomycin, as a last resort, one can turn to prayer. The patient kneels down and prays that the warts go away, and the physician kneels down and prays that the patient goes away.

The bottom line in the treatment of warts is that you win some and you lose some. There is no one way to treat a wart. You can try every treatment you can think of and you may still fail. It is indeed a humbling experience.

CHAPTER V

"The Psyche and the Skin"

It is well known that the psyche may affect the responses in the skin through the vasculature and the nerve endings. For example, in a frightful event there is the saying that, he turned white with fear or she paled when she heard the bad news. In embarrassment he or she turned red and blushed furiously. Sometimes something you see or think makes your hair stand on end or makes your skin crawl.

When I was an intern, the attending dermatologist would conduct an outpatient dermatology clinic at the hospital. The nurse would ready the patient for presentation. Dermatology residents would answer the questions the attending would ask. The interns would write the prescriptions. The medical students and nurses were there to see, listen, and learn. On one occasion, the nurse brought in a vagrant who was literally crawling with pubic lice. The attending dermatologist asked questions regarding the louse phthirus pubis. Did it travel elsewhere, for example, to the eyelashes? How long had the lice been present if you examined the

nit on the hair shaft? What did the nit feel like?

What insecticides were to be used to kill the louse?

How do you to get rid of the nits by either plucking

or shaving the hair, etc?

That night my wife awakened me and said,

"What are you doing? You're scratching like

crazy."

Indeed, I was, and in my dreams, I thought

I felt the lice crawling on my skin, and I was

scratching in my sleep.

An occasional patient will complain of itching

of the scalp. It might be real or imagined, but I

always look for head lice and feel for nits on the hair shaft as the cause of an itchy scalp.

A wise dermatologist once said, "If the diagnosis does not quite fit that of a known diagnosis, consider the diagnoses of an insect bite, a facticial lesion, or a drug reaction."

DELUSIONS OF PARASITOSIS:

Patients may come to the dermatologist complaining that they have bugs crawling on their skin. They will come in with envelopes containing brown and black specks that they have collected. Examining these under a microscope show only bits of skin and dried blood.

After explaining to such a patient that no bugs were present, I then referred him to a psychiatrist who might be able to help him. The next morning in the local paper was an article about a man who had doused himself with gasoline and burned himself to death. He apparently felt that burning his skin was the only way to rid himself of his bugs.

THE HOTEL ITCH: A number of years ago a man and his son stayed at a hotel in Iowa. The next day, he came in with lesions that looked like insect bites. I asked him if he had been in the hot tub. Occasionally, hot tubs will contain bacteria that can cause papular urticaria in some patients. He said that he had been in the hot tub, but his daughter had not been in the hot tub, and she had these bites. Finally, I called the manager of the hotel and told him that one of the residents who had stayed there had gotten insect bites, and I wondered if any pets had slept on the beds. He denied this. Then I asked him if they had any insects that they knew about. They said that the hotel was located near the river, and at that time of the year, sand flies were coming through the screening on the windows. They were particularly bad that summer, and they were biting those staying at the hotel. I termed this bizarre case "The Hotel Itch." Think of insect bites when a diagnosis doesn't fit.

THE CASE OF THE JILTED LOVER:

A young man who was living with his girlfriend got into an argument with her and he moved out. After returning to his own apartment, he came in to see me with insect bites. They were most likely bed bug bites, as bed bugs bite in sets of three (breakfast, lunch, and dinner). He felt that he had hives because he had left his girlfriend. In fact, after he had gone back to his own apartment, he was being bitten by the bed bugs in his apartment.

He was told that if he would turn on the lights in the middle of the night and look in the creases in the mattress or on the frame of the bed, he would find bed bugs. He did so and they were there. The cause of his hives were found.

THE ANIMAL LOVER: Many patients sleep with their dogs and cats. A man came in with generalized urticaria. He denied taking any medications or over-the-counter drugs. Short courses of prednisone did not help him. When questioned, he insisted that his cat did not have fleas. I asked him if he could possibly sleep without the cat for one week to see if the hives would disappear. He said that he could do this for a week, but he didn't know if the cat could, as he said that the cat would meow all night long scratching at the door. He said that he would try this. After a week, he had no hives. Still he would not give up his cat. We settled on the compromise of letting the cat sleep at the foot of the bed, but not on or in the bed.

Many times the cats or dogs will have left the house for one reason or another. The fleas then have no one to bite as the natural hosts are gone. They then attack humans. Also that is why when pets are brought into hotels or motels and the guests leave, sometimes the fleas are left behind on the bedspread. Another guest comes along and will be bitten by the fleas on the bedspread. If the pet is no longer in the home and if one sits on the chair or couch where the pet usually sits, then the fleas will attack the humans.

Edward S. Peterka MD MS

THE SEVEN YEAR ITCH: One of the difficult cases to diagnose may be scabies, sometimes termed the seven-year itch. The mite Sarcoptes scabiei is the cause. The mite burrows in the layers of the skin between the interdigital spaces. The feces of the mite or a body part of the mite causes the inflammation and itching. Putting an ink drop in the interdigital space may be used to detect the burrough. Skin scrapings or a biopsy may reveal the mite or the body parts of the mite. Treatment with insecticides, such as one percent Lindane lotion, or shampoos with five percent Permethrin, will kill the mite. One must observe care in treating pregnant women and infants.

A number of years ago a woman was seen in consultation for her chronic eczema. She had been treated with topical and systemic steroids. These helped relieve the itching, but she never completely cleared. Scrapings showed Sarcoptes scabiei in the interdigital spaces. She was treated with six percent precipitated sulfur in a cream base which resulted in a cure. Occasionally, a patient will have been treated for scabies and will continue to have itching in the interdigital spaces and palms. This is called post-scabetic syndrome. Treatment with topical steroids and six percent precipitated sulfur cream for a period of time will often relieve the condition.

One of the worst type of insect bites is the brown recluse spider bite. This spider bite is painless, but the venom causes a severe necrotic reaction. The brown spider lives under porches, sheds, and in barns. The venomous necrotic reaction becomes a surgical problem and requires immediate treatment. Black widow spider bites, on the other hand, are painful. The black widow spider can be identified by the red dot on its back. The venom is also necrotizing.

Lyme Disease, first described in Lyme, Connecticut is caused by the deer tick. These ticks transmit the spirochete Borrelia burgdorfari through the tick bite. A skin sign is the red macular annular lesion on the skin following the tick bite. If untreated, neurological and arthritic symptoms may occur at a later date. Insect bites become infected locally and the infection must be treated.

An elderly woman was convinced that she had pain in her forehead and to get it out, she was going to cut it out with a razor blade. She kept cutting her forehead with a razor inflicting cuts that would never heal. I convinced her to see a psychiatrist.

The third leg of the stool when the diagnoses does not quite fit is an unusual drug reaction. Drug reactions may cause a large variety of symptoms and dermatology books have chapters on the skin manifestations of drug reactions. There may be fixed drug eruptions, drugs that cause photosensitivity, drugs that induce systemic lupus erythematosus, and drugs that cause a host of other reactions.

If the diagnosis does not quite fit, consider the diagnoses of insect bites, facticial lesions, or drug reactions.

CHAPTER VI

"Longevity"

An elderly patient came into my office one day. I looked at his chart and I said to him,

"Are you really 98 years old?"

"Yes," he said, "I'm the oldest living farmer in the state of Illinois."

"Are you still farming?" I asked.

"Yes," he said, I was on the <u>Johnny Carson Show</u>."

"What was he like?" I asked.

"Oh, he was a pretty nice fellow. I told him I had a 65-year-old girlfriend. He teased me about robbing the cradle."

"What else did he ask you?" I said.

He asked me, "To what do you attribute your longevity?"

"What did you tell him?" I asked.

"I told him that, I guess I was just made out of the right stuff," he said.

I think he was right. Much of a person's longevity is his genes.

Another gentleman came in my office one day. I noticed on the chart that he was 80 years old. He didn't look a day over 65.

"How is it that you look so young?" I asked him.

"It's the fresh air," he said.

"What do you mean?" I said to him.

"Well, when my wife and I first got married, we made an agreement. If we had an argument, she would go into the kitchen and I would go outside. I guess it's all those years of fresh air that has kept me young," he replied.

This reminds me of the lady who remarked about the golden years, "The only thing golden about the golden years is your teeth are yellow and your pee is yellow."

Stress is a significant factor in longevity. Healthy living leads to healthy skin. Stress will lead to ulcers, nail biting, picking, overeating and smoking.

Stress is a two-way street. People stress you and you stress people.

Certainly, a good outlook with humor helps. It has been said that a good belly laugh uses up 80 calories. A jellyroll will lead to a bellyroll. Pushing away from the table is sometimes the best exercise. Sugar has more calories and is fattening. The key is a balance somewhere in between.

I often go to meetings where I meet old friends. One of the first things I ask is, "What's new?"

A friend of mine who was elderly said, " I just got married."

"Oh, was she rich?" I asked.

" No, she wasn't rich. She wasn't poor either. She was sort of in between," he said.

"Was she young?" I asked.

"No," she wasn't young, and she wasn't old," he said, "She was sort of in between."

"She must have been very beautiful," I then said.

"No," he said. "She wasn't beautiful, but she wasn't homely either. She was sort of in between."

I then asked him, "Why did you marry her?"

"Because she can drive at night," he said. He could no longer drive at night because of his loss of night vision.

During the Great Depression after the stockmarket crashed in 1929, when I was a young boy, my mother would say to me, "Eat your carrots. They are good for your eyes!" That was before Vitamin A or Beta-Carotene was ever thought of as being necessary for night vision.

There is a story of two University of Illinois professors who tried to grow two fields of corn on the farm campus near the stadium to represent the colors of the university. One field would be blue and the other field would be orange. Instead, they got a cross between blue and orange that was a muddy brown color. They discovered that the corn was rich in beta-carotene or Vitamin A. In the rice bowl countries at that time, there was much loss of night vision from lack of Vitamin A in their diet. The scientists urged these countries to grow the Vitamin A rich corn, which they did, and the corn was put into their diet. This cured their loss of night vision. A proper balanced diet is one of the keys to longevity.

CHAPTER VII

"The Aging Skin"

If you live long enough, you too, will someday grow old. Change is the one constant in a changing world. As a person ages, certain hair and skin changes take place. Men tend to lose their hair in an inverted "M" pattern or a bald spot appears on the back of the head. In women, there is thinning of the hair in female type pattern baldness. A woman's big concern is if she will get bald. The answer is no. Women do not become bald, but their hair in general becomes thinner. Telogen effluvium, alopecia areata, and post-partem hair loss must be differentiated from female pattern baldness.

If there is a history of long sun exposure, in later years the face may begin to show signs of sun damage. The skin becomes leathery and wrinkled. In our present day culture women want a beautiful, deep tan. They spend more and more time in the sun or in a tanning booth to achieve this. What they don't realize is that their skin will later become dry, wrinkled, and leathery and they will get actinic keratoses and skin cancers years later.

In the late eighteenth and early nineteenth centuries, women protected their skin by parasols, long sleeves, and high neck dresses. If they were wealthy, they avoided the sun. Only mad dogs and Englishmen went out in the midday sun. An elderly man or woman who earlier had spent years working in an outdoor garden, working on a farm, or working as a sailor will show sun damaged skin later in life The areas of unexposed skin are smooth and white like a baby's skin.

As people age, they have more cardiovascular accidents or strokes. In Parkinson's disease, as in stroke, the skin becomes oily and greasy with increased seborrhea and flaking of the scalp. As a person ages, Herpes zoster or "shingles" are more severe than in children or younger adults. Herpes zoster of the second trigeminal nerve may involve the eyes and lead to corneal scarring if it is not treated aggressively. Systemic steroids and antiviral medication in high doses may prevent the eye complications or the post zoster neuralgia which defy all treatment. Neurologists offer some relief from the pain and discomfort with certain drugs.

An occasional patient will experience pain in the area of the first trigeminal nerve either the right or left scalp without showing the classical blistering of "shingles". A course of antiviral medications may relieve the symptoms. One must be aware that temporal arteritis may mimic the neuralgic pain of Herpes zoster.

As people age, they lose some moles and get new ones. As people age, they find that they must take more medications for diseases such as heart disease, hypertension, and other conditions. Some specialists deal only in diseases of the elderly (i.e. geriatric medicine). In older men, the incidence of benign prostatic hypertrophy and cancer of the prostate is much higher than in younger men. Because of this, older men have urgency and frequency and ask, "Where is the nearest bathroom?"

Elderly patients handle general anesthesia poorly. In general, they do not handle six or seven medications without experiencing drug interaction.

A patient came in complaining about her family physician. She told me that her doctor had told her that she would have to take medication for her high blood pressure for the rest of her life.

"Well," I said "that sometimes happens."

"Yes," she exclaimed, "but he only gave me five pills!"

As people age and if they have had years of sun exposure, melanoma becomes more common. It is directly related to the years of sun exposure. Many older persons have dark freckles or sunspots called senile lentigines, not because the patients are senile, but because they have more freckles and dark spots. Then the question becomes which dark spot is malignant? One looks for the one flower that stands out in a garden of flowers. Skin cancers are especially common in persons with blue eyes and blonde hair and those with reddish complexions. African Americans who have pigmented skin rarely get skin cancers. They get other diseases unique to their race, but skin cancer is not one of them. A person's occupation, such as a line man, a farmer, or a sailor with years of exposure to ultraviolet light from the sun have a higher incidence of skin cancers. Years later, they come in with numerous actinic keratoses that are premalignant lesions or with skin cancers.

In general, when seeing either young or old patients, but especially older patients, follow this pattern. Examine the patient, listen to the patient, and consider the possibilities. Be a possibility thinker and ask questions.

The last question that I always ask the patient after explaining the diagnosis and treatment is, "Do you have any questions?"

ABOUT THE AUTHOR

Dr. Peterka received a Bachelor of Arts degree in Interdepartmental Studies from the University of Minnesota in Minneapolis, Minnesota with minors in philosophy, history, mathematics, physics, and abnormal psychology graduating Magna Cum Laude and Phi Beta Kappa. He received a Bachelor of Science Degree in 1958. In his senior year in medical school he studied dermatology under Doctors Francis Lynch, Henry Michelson, and Robert Goltz. He earned his M.D. degree from the University of Minnesota Medical School in Minneapolis in 1961.

In 1962 he interned at Ancker General Hospital in St. Paul, Minnesota and in 1963 began his dermatology residency in the Department of Dermatology University of Minnesota Hospitals. During his residency he studied porphyrin abnormalities with Dr. Cecil Watson and did studies on red blood cell hemolysis and pathology of the skin in erythropoetic protoporphyria and sun sensitivity. He studied sun sensitivity in American Indians at the Indian Reservation in Red Lake, Minnesota. He received a Master of Science Degree from the University of Minnesota, Minneapolis, Minnesota writing his thesis on <u>Cutaneous Carbohydrate Studies</u>. He was involved with skin testing of prisoners at the Minnesota State Prison, Stillwater, Minnesota for Minnesota Mining and Manufacturing (3M) testing their various types of tapes for skin sensitivity. He worked as an assistant professor in the Division of Dermatology at the University of Colorado Medical School from 1965 to 1968 teaching medical residents in dermatology and pediatrics.

In 1968 he moved to Galesburg, Illinois to practice dermatology. He joined the Dermatology Department as clinical associate professor at the Abraham Lincoln School of Medicine, Chicago, Illinois teaching medical students and residents. In 1968 he became the first head of the Department of

Dermatology at Peoria School of Medicine, Peoria, Illinois and gave weekly lectures to the medical staff and residents in family practice at Methodist Hospital, Peoria, Illinois.

Dr. Peterka enjoys fishing, writing, and inventing. He is an officer of Rotary International and is a Past Grand Knight in the Knights of Columbus. He is a charter member of the Spoon River Mental Health Association and a charter member of the Illinois Dermatological Society. His interests are books and literature on Abraham Lincoln and he has written a paper on the skin lesions of Abraham Lincoln. He enjoys and collects stories and jokes and has written a joke book "Laughter Is the Best

Medicine or the Surly Bird Gets the Germ". He has been President of Knox County Medical Society and a delegate to the Illinois State Medical Society.

He married his wife Jean when a junior in medical school, and after 45 years of marriage, they have five children and six grandchildren.

www.ingramcontent.com/pod-product-compliance
Lightning Source LLC
Chambersburg PA
CBHW022102170526
45157CB00004B/1453